DO I LOOK ~~FAT~~ GREAT IN THESE JEANS?

INSIDER'S GUIDE TO COSMETIC SURGERY

Dr. John Gonzalez
FACS, FAACS, FACOG

ISBN-13: 978-1717131218
ISBN-10: 1717131212

Thank you to my wife Leonor, my son David, and my daughter Catherine for their support on this journey to write a book. I also want to thank, my partner, Dr. Michelle Owens for always having my back and my nephew Danny for pushing me to be a better man.

The information in this book is not intended or implied to be a substitute for professional medical advice, diagnosis or treatment. All content, including text, graphics, images and information, in this book is for general information purposes only. You are encouraged to confirm any information obtained from or through this book with other sources and review all information regarding any medical condition or treatment with your physician.

NEVER DISREGARD PROFESSIONAL MEDICAL ADVICE OR DELAY SEEKING MEDICAL TREATMENT BECAUSE OF SOMETHING YOU HAVE READ IN THIS BOOK

TABLE OF CONTENTS

Chapter 1

Let's Get Started!

I wrote this book for those patients who are ready to act and begin to feel better about their bodies. It is an opportunity for you to get inside the mind of a cosmetic surgeon who has been helping people just like you realize their dreams and improve their self-image.

At the time of this book writing, I have performed approximately twelve to thirteen hundred cosmetic breast surgery cases, a few hundred liposuction cases, and over 100 tummy tucks. In June of 2017, we moved into our new 9500 square foot AAAHC accredited facility to better serve our patients and it is our goal to be the leading provider of women's health in South Louisiana.

I began my practice in 1999 and I am board certified in Obstetrics and Gynecology, as well as Female Pelvic Medicine and Reconstructive Surgery. I first became interested in cosmetic surgery back in 2006 when I was looking to expand some of the services offered to our patients.

Since my original training was in obstetrics and gynecology, I have been performing surgery for a long time and I have delivered a couple thousand babies. At the time of a cesarean section or hysterectomy, I would have a lot of patients say, "Doc, while you are there can you go ahead and tighten up my muscles or suck out some of that fat?", so it just came to be a natural progression for my practice to start offering cosmetic services.

I spent a lot of time studying alternative and less invasive ways to do surgery. Cosmetic surgery had come so far in 2006 but it still seemed as though most people were still having to undergo general anesthesia to have these procedures.

I came across tumescent anesthesia, which is something that we are going to talk a great deal about a little bit later in the book. That was the real impetus for starting this journey 12 years ago. Tumescent anesthesia is a form of local anesthesia where patients do not have to go to sleep to have their cosmetic procedures.

There were doctors in California and in the northeast, who were beginning to publish papers describing their techniques. It was not long after that I became a student of their work and received training in their technique.

I was fascinated by the idea of performing surgery on patients without having to put them to sleep or enduring all of the risks associated with general anesthesia.

Cosmetic surgery is much more common than it was just a decade ago and chances are you know many people who have had these types of procedures (even if they haven't shared it with you).

According to the American Society of Plastic Surgeons, the top 5 cosmetic surgeries performed in the United States are breast augmentations, rhinoplasty (nose reshaping), eyelid surgeries, liposuction, and tummy tucks.

In our practice, we focus mainly on cosmetic body procedures where we do breast augmentations, breast lifts, breast reductions, liposuction with or without fat transfer, and tummy tucks.

Question 1

According to the American Society of Aesthetic Plastic Surgery.

Which of the following is NOT one of the top five cosmetic surgeries performed in 2017?

a. Nose reshaping
b. Face lift
c. Breast augmentation
d. Liposuction
e. Eyelid surgery
f. Abdominoplasty (Tummy Tuck)

The answer is b. A face lift was not in the top five of all cosmetic procedures performed in 2017.

Chapter 2

Is Cosmetic Surgery Right for Me?

That is a great question, and, really, is a question that only YOU can answer. I mean there are some things that can preclude you from having cosmetic surgery. If you have certain health conditions, then you may not be a good candidate for elective cosmetic surgery. But in general, if it is right for you, depends on the reasons you want surgery.

I make sure to ask my patients the reason they want a cosmetic procedure and what do they expect to look like after surgery. Some common answers I have received when I have asked my patients "WHY" they want surgery are:

"I am done having children and just want my breasts to be higher and fuller and want to fit better in my clothes."

"I have been small chested my entire life and now I can finally afford to get breast implants."

"For my entire adult life, I have put my family's needs before my own and now it is time to take care of me!".

What is your reason for having cosmetic surgery? Think about it and come up with an answer before even making an appointment for a consultation. I can tell you there are some answers that are a RED FLAG for me. These answers include:

"I want to fix my relationship my husband."

"I have tried everything else to lose weight and just can't."

"I want to look like (type your favorite movie star or model's name here)."

Once you have answered why you want cosmetic surgery and what type of outcome you are expecting, call our office at (337) 785-2006 to make an appointment for a free consultation so we can go over things and get you started on your way to unlocking the new YOU.

Am I too old for cosmetic surgery?

The truth is that there are no age limits to having cosmetic surgery. I have done breast augmentations on women in their 70s. I have done liposuction and fat transfers on women in their 60s and 70s, as well. So, in other words, every case is individualized.

It will depend on the type of surgery, how extensive the surgery, as well as that person's medical history. In other words, do not let your age hold you back from calling our office for a consultation appointment.

Who is a good candidate for cosmetic surgery?

Well, I can tell you that there are many factors which need to be considered to determine who is a good candidate for surgery. But for the purpose of this book I want to focus on things that you have control over.

First and foremost, it is important that you have realistic expectations. I always get a little nervous when patients come up to me and present photographs of people that they want to look like.

They will say "Oh I want my butt to look like this" or "I want breasts like this" or "I want to make sure I am as thin as this person," and a lot of times, depending on where we are starting from, some of those results may not be obtainable.

So, I try to make sure that I listen well to my patients and make sure we have a good dialogue about setting realistic expectations.

Another factor is whether or not a patient is a smoker. We know that nonsmokers are better candidates for cosmetic surgery than smokers. That doesn't mean you can't have cosmetic surgery if you are a smoker, but smoking would increase certain risks and complications both during surgery, as well as during the postoperative healing period.

Most patients who smoke do just fine, but whenever there is an unexpected or less than ideal outcome from cosmetic surgery, that patient is usually a smoker. Though I am not a smoker, I have many family members who smoke and realize it is not easy to quit.

I try and encourage patients who smoke to quit at least two to three weeks before surgery and at least six to eight weeks after surgery.

Whether or not you have certain medical problems, may also play a role in determining if you are a good surgical candidate. If you are a poorly controlled diabetic or hypertensive, it would make you a higher risk candidate for cosmetic surgery.

If you have ever had a deep vein thrombosis, DVT, or pulmonary embolism, known as PE, we would most likely not consider you a candidate for any surgery that was not medically necessary.

For most patients, this is something that is individualized, and we would go over with you at the time of your consultation.

What effect can cosmetic surgery have on my self-image?

It is pretty amazing the difference I see in patients when they have had cosmetic surgery. Remember, I delivered babies for many years and I have been blessed to be part of some of the happiest moments in many people's lives. But there is nothing like the joy a patient receives when they finally have that breast augmentation or liposuction of that muffin top they have been trying to get rid of for years.

Many women describe it is a different type of joy. They describe it to me as a feeling of finally doing something for themselves.

Let me tell you a little story about a patient who came to see me when I first started performing breast augmentations in 2007. When I asked her why she wanted to have breast implants, I remember her mentioning to me that she was very self-conscious about the appearance of her breasts.

She went on to tell me that every time she was intimate with her husband she would make sure the lights were off or she had her shirt on.

That was something that really stuck with me, because it made me feel so bad for her. I ended up doing her breast augmentation surgery and she had a great result.

The funny thing is about two months later I had another patient who came to speak with me, and she said "Dr. Gonzalez! I don't know if you realize this, but there is a woman in the waiting room who lifted her shirt and is showing someone her breasts. They are out there for everyone to see." Needless to say, I was startled by this news.

After I did a little investigating to see what was going on, it just so happened that the patient who originally was self-conscious, so much that even during intimacy with her husband would hide her breasts, had now ended up being TOO comfortable. She was showing people who were coming in to see me for a consultation, what I great job I had done.

In the matter of a few months, she went from self-conscious in front of her own husband, to flashing strangers in a public waiting room. I can't promise that if you have cosmetic surgery too you will be as happy as she was because the experience is different, and everyone has their own reactions, but in my experience most patients will feel much better about their body and it will improve their self-image.

Can someone be addicted to cosmetic surgery?

When I think of addiction, I usually think of alcohol or drugs. To many people in the medical profession, addiction refers to something that is habit forming and will result in severe trauma if the substance or thing is withheld.

So, in that sense, I will tell you no cosmetic surgery is non- addictive. However, there are some patients who might take it a little too far and look for an easy way out. It may give them the feeling that cosmetic surgery can make them feel good about themselves. Those are the patients we watch out for.

We try to make sure we are doing surgery for the right reasons and on the right patients, but sometimes, it is difficult. Some patients "Doctor Shop" and aren't always truthful about all the cosmetic surgeries that they have had or withhold information on their medical history.

So, in essence, cosmetic surgery is not addictive but there are some patients that can push the limits of cosmetic surgery and put themselves at risk for potential harm and/or, even possibly, a poor outcome.

Will this fix my relationship with my partner?

One time, I had a couple who were having a lot of marital difficulties and the woman said that she wanted a tummy tuck.

Like I usually do during my consultations, I asked her why she wanted surgery and what kind of result was she expecting. Her response broke my heart.

She went on to tell me her husband wanted her to do the surgery because he was not physically attracted to her anymore since she had their three children. Needless to say, we had a very long discussion about surgery not fixing anyone's relationship and I referred them both to marriage counseling.

I wish I could tell you this was an isolated occurrence, but the truth is I have run into many patients who turn to cosmetic surgery to try and fix a troubled relationship or to make themselves more attractive to their partners.

My answer is always the same. If anyone is having relationship problems, they should talk and communicate with their partner, and consider getting counseling.

The last thing you want to do is have cosmetic surgery. Marriage counseling can be expensive, but the money is better spent seeing a therapist to help both partners get through their difficulties.

What should I do to achieve the best results from cosmetic surgery?

If I had to answer that question in one simple phrase it would be "follow your doctor's instructions". I can't tell you how often I counsel patients about no lifting anything heavier than five to ten pounds after surgery. When they come to see me four days later for their post op visit, they are holding their baby carrier with their twenty-five-pound baby in it.

Now, I understand there are some obligations you have and not everyone is able to limit their physical activity, but patients must understand that if they do not follow the advice that we provide, then they are setting themselves up for complications and problems healing.

Another thing that can be done to achieve the best results is to be patient and let things heal. People often expect to see the final result immediately after surgery. I spend a lot of time informing patients that there is often a lot of swelling shortly after surgery and we will not be able to judge the results for some time. This is particularly true for cosmetic breast surgery.

Implants are often high and look squarish after surgery. It takes up to two to six weeks to finally look more normal and can take up to four to six months for implants to finally settle into their permanent place.

One of the things I go over with every patient having cosmetic surgery is the fact that many women can suffer from worsening depression or anxiety after surgery. I quote on my consent form that about 30% of women get extremely anxious after surgery and start to obsess over the results and begin to regret their decision.

I explain to them that once the swelling goes down and we have a better idea of the final results the anxiety usually goes away.

Other things that you can do to optimize your outcome is to not smoke. I cannot tell you how many times we have a postoperative healing issue or infection and when

I look back into their medical history, the patient always seems to be a smoker.

I encourage you to please be honest with your doctor. We recognize that smoking is an addiction and it is difficult to quit smoking but ask your doctor for help and postpone your surgery if you are having trouble quitting. Anything you can do to quit or minimize your use of tobacco before surgery and during the first few months healing will help.

Most smokers do just fine and do not have any complications with surgery, but everyone must understand the risks of certain complications are higher in those who smoke.

Another thing you can do to give yourself the best chance of healing is to watch your pain medications. Patients tend to think they have to be "pain free" after surgery. This is just not true. The purpose of pain medication is to make pain manageable. I will tell you that recovering from most surgeries can be very uncomfortable.

I do not recommend overdoing pain medication and only take it as prescribed by your doctor. Do not EVER use anyone else's pain medicine and never share your medicine with others. Taking too much pain medicine can lead to addiction, severe bloating with constipation, and over sedation.

Question 2

True or False

Having liposuction is a great way to lose weight?

False. Liposuction is a great way to decrease the size of fatty deposits, but it is a poor way to lose weight.

Chapter 3

What's the Difference Between Cosmetic and Plastic Surgery?

Cosmetic and plastic surgery are terms often used interchangeably by many people. However, they are not the same. Not all cosmetic surgeons are plastic surgeons and not all plastic surgeons are cosmetic surgeons.

Cosmetic surgery is a discipline of medicine that focuses on enhancing features. In other words, improving features and trying to make people look better.

As opposed to plastic surgery which is mainly focused on repairing the defects people have and to restore the normal function or appearance of something. Plastic surgeons are fantastic surgeons when it comes to facial fractures after trauma, repairing cleft palates, or reconstructing a breast after breast cancer surgery, but cosmetic surgery requires a different level of expertise.

What is the difference in training in a plastic and cosmetic surgeon?

The first thing to realize is that there is no residency program specifically focused on cosmetic surgery. As a matter of fact, there are many cosmetic surgeons from a variety of different medical specialties.

It is not uncommon for a gynecologic surgeon or a general surgeon to have received additional training in breast or body cosmetic procedures. ENT's, oral/maxillofacial surgeons, and ophthalmologists often perform facial cosmetic surgeries. All of this training is done after a traditional residency program.

The same can be said for most plastic surgeons. The vast majority of their residency training is actually done in reconstructive surgery. They receive a lot of hand surgery training and burn reconstructive surgeries. So, their residency program specifically focused on the reconstructive aspects of surgery.

Many plastic surgeons feel the need to obtain additional training in cosmetic surgery after completing their plastic surgery residency and many times receive this training from non-plastic surgery training programs.

I realize all of this can be confusing.

The important thing to know is that the field of cosmetic surgery is not solely confined to any one specialty. There are plastic surgeons who would like you to believe that they are the only ones qualified to perform cosmetic surgery. Nothing can be further from the truth.

No one medical specialty owns the field of cosmetic surgery.

The Father of Modern Liposuction

For example, when we look at liposuction, we know that **Doctor Giorgio Fischer, who was an Italian gynecologist**, was the first person to invent the blunt cannula used during liposuction to create tunnels which allows fat to be sucked out easily and safer than prior methods.

It is important to note, Dr. Fischer was not a plastic surgeon, yet he is widely recognized as a pioneer in one of the most common cosmetic surgeries performed.

Who discovered the cosmetic use for Botox?

If you guessed it was a plastic surgeon, then, you answered incorrectly.

Botox is used to help smooth out facial wrinkles and the interesting thing is that the two doctors, Drs. Jean and

Alastair Carruthers, who discovered the cosmetic uses for Botox (botulism toxin) in 1987 were ophthalmologist.

They were originally using the toxin to treat the uncontrollable blinking and spasming of the eye and surrounding areas, a medical condition called blepharospasm.

To their surprise, patients began asking it to be injected in their foreheads because it would make the wrinkles on their foreheads go away. It was not long after when other areas of the face were being injected with the toxin to smooth out wrinkles and, as they say, the "rest is history"

Who came up with tumescent anesthesia?

Another physician who has made a great contribution to cosmetic surgery is Dr. Jeffrey Klein. Dr. Klein is a dermatologist and was very interested in liposuction.

He realized that everyone was having liposuction under general anesthesia and were having excessive amounts of blood loss during the procedure. The amount of fat removed was actually limited by the amount of blood that was lost during the surgery.

Dr. Klein came up with a dilute solution which allowed the surgeon to perform liposuction under tumescent anesthesia, a form of local anesthesia, where a patient does not have to go to sleep.

He also included in his solution a compound known as epinephrine which also addressed the bleeding issues, allowing for a minimal amount of blood loss during the procedure.

Since then, other pioneers have made modifications to Dr. Klein's Solution and now use it to perform breast augmentations and tummy tucks.

In this chapter, we have learned that three of the largest contributions to the field of cosmetic medicine have been made by a gynecologist, two ophthalmologists and a dermatologist.

So, the next time you are in our office getting Botox, having liposuction, or about to undergo a breast augmentation under local anesthesia, say a quiet thanks to these medical innovators.

Question 3

What surgeries can Dr. Gonzalez perform in his accredited in-office operating room suite?

a. Breast augmentation
b. Liposuction
c. Brazilian Butt Lift
d. Brazilian Tummy Tuck
e. All of the Above

The answer is e. We can perform all of the procedures in our in-office accredited operating room suite under local anesthesia

Chapter 4

Choosing a Cosmetic Surgeon

What questions should I ask during my consultation?

There are a lot of different things to consider when deciding who is going to be your cosmetic surgeon. The first thing I would tell you is to let others know you are planning to have cosmetic surgery and ask friends and family who they recommend.

You will be surprised to find out how many people you didn't know have had some of these procedures. The more people you ask the more likely the same surgeon's name will come up.

In my practice, about 70% of our new patients come as referrals from other patients. That is an amazing statistic and means we have a lot of happy patients. As a matter of fact, it is not uncommon in my practice for a husband or boyfriend of a patient we have performed surgery on, to talk to his buddies and the next thing you know, their wives and girlfriends are coming to see me for a consultation.

How do I contact you "after hours" if I am having problems or questions?

This may not be on the top of most people's list of questions, but I will tell you, in no uncertain term, it is vital.

There are many issues which come up after hours and cannot wait until the morning or Monday. I give all my cosmetic surgery patients my personal cell phone number.

I am available to my patients 24 hours a day, 7 days a week. If I have cellphone service, I can be reached by my patients. I answer my phone and text messages even on vacation.

<u>Yes, it is important to have a work- life balance, but I want my patients to know they can reach me when they need me.</u>

Do you have before and after photos?

If I was going to have a cosmetic surgery procedure, I would most definitely ask to see before and after photos. I would, specifically, ask if the photos presented to me are their work.

There are some surgeons known to take photographs from other websites and claim them to be their own. I often tell my patients that their surgical outcome typically depends on where they are starting from.

Try and request before and after photographs of people who have some of your same measurements, so you can get a better idea of what your outcome may be. Most cosmetic surgeons place photos of patients who are of ideal weight and body frame on their websites or photo albums, but people come in all shapes and sizes.

If you are six feet tall and weigh one-hundred thirty pounds, your postoperative outcome most likely will not be the same as someone five-foot-tall weighing one-hundred thirty pounds.

How many of these have you performed?

It is intuitive to think the more of any one procedure a surgeon performs, the better they will be at that particular surgery.

If you are considering a breast augmentation, finding a cosmetic surgeon who has a lot of experience placing implants is a must. Also asking how many they do per month or per year will give you insight into a surgeon's experience.

For example, I can tell you since ***I began doing breast augmentations in 2007, I have probably done around over 1200-1300 cosmetic breast surgery cases. If we look at the last 4 years, I have done over 800, or an average of 200 breast cases a year.*** I think you will have a hard time finding anybody who has had that extensive experience. There may be a handful of surgeons who do that many cases a year, but the vast majority of cosmetic surgeons will perform less.

So, what is the right number of surgeries you should feel comfortable with? That would be hard to say. However, in my opinion, if you see a doctor who is doing less than 50 breast augmentations a year, you should consider choosing someone who does them more frequently.

Where will my surgery be performed?

Cosmetic surgery can be performed in many different surgical settings. Sometimes surgery can take place in a hospital, an ambulatory surgical center, or it can be performed in an office operating room. Where a surgeon chooses to do your procedure depends on many factors.

In our practice, we do the vast majority of our cosmetic surgeries in our office operating room. Our facility has two operating room suites where we do our surgeries under local or tumescent anesthesia. However, we do have some cases that require different levels of anesthesia than we can provide in our office, so we do those in a hospital setting.

No matter where the surgeon chooses to do your surgery, the most important question to ask is if that facility is accredited. The three main accrediting bodies who inspect and review operating room facilities are Joint Commission, JCAHO, Accreditation Association for Ambulatory Health Care, AAAHC, and American Association for Accreditation of Ambulatory Surgical Facilities, AAAASF.

All these organizations will inspect the facility to make sure policies and procedures are in place to assure patient safety. Once a facility is accredited, it is usually good for three years.

Even though accreditation has been confirmed, these agencies sometimes make surprise visits to make sure all standards are being met. You need to make sure that your surgery is performed in an accredited facility.

We pride ourselves on having our office accredited by AAAHC. It has undergone numerous inspections and has always managed to maintain its certification.

What does it mean to be board certified?

The first thing to understand is that board certification and having a medical license are not the same thing. To get a medical license, you have to meet minimum education and training criteria in the state where a doctor practices. The state will, then, grant the doctor a medical license.

Board certification is a voluntary process a physician goes through to demonstrate an expertise in a particular specialty or subspecialty.

I cannot stress enough to you that finding a board-certified doctor is very important. But remember, there is no universally accepted board-certification in cosmetic surgery.

Now, a plastic surgeon may tell you that you should only see a board-certified plastic surgeon. I will go so far to tell you that I think being board certified in one of the surgical specialties is important, but equally important is the training a surgeon has received after residency in cosmetic surgery.

Being board certified will give you some assurance they are qualified in their primary specialty but won't necessarily translate to their competence in performing your cosmetic procedure.

I am board certified by the American Board of Obstetrics and Gynecology in both Obstetrics and Gynecology, as well as, Female Pelvic Medicine and Reconstructive Surgery. In addition, I have received specialized training in cosmetic surgery.

What makes you qualified to do cosmetic surgery?

We can go over my education, training and experience again to prove how I am qualified to do cosmetic surgery. However, I think the fact that you have reached this point in the book, possibly shows you already know all that.

Instead, let me tell you a little more about me. I grew up in a home full of women. My father was not involved much in my life.

As a matter of fact, I do not have any memories of him at all. My mother had three children. I have two older sisters and I am the baby of the family. I have been around women my entire life.

If you are from the south, you may relate to this story. There are often get-togethers where the women spend the evening hovered in one room socializing, while the men are all having fun in another room. Well I am the one man always next to my wife in the women's group.

If we ever play *Battle of the Sexes* as the game for Family Game Night, the women NEVER let me play on the men's team because I know too many of their answers. I have been relegated to a lonesome chair where the team members can "PHONE- A- JOHN'. I understand women. I am a good listener and, apparently, I speak "Women".

What are my options if I am unhappy with the results?

I think something to discuss during your consultation is if there are going to be charges should you require revisional surgery. In most cases, if there is a revision surgery, there probably will be some additional charges, which you will be responsible.

Most cosmetic surgeons I know will keep the cost to a minimum and usually just charge you the cost of the procedure and not for their time. However, it is important to understand there is a difference between not having a perfect outcome and having an unacceptable outcome.

Most of the time if a patient has been properly counseled and has reasonable expectations this isn't usually an issue.

Like I tell all my cosmetic breast surgery patients during my consultations "we are not making twins, we are just trying to make pretty close sisters."

How many consultations should I get before scheduling?

You will read online that getting many different consultations before deciding on a surgeon is a good idea. I would never discourage someone from getting multiple consultations but sometimes too many opinions can often lead to a lot of confusion and make it more difficult to make a decision.

In my experience, for most routine consultations such as a breast augmentation, tummy tuck or liposuction, it really comes down to how the surgeon made you feel during your consultation. Are they a good listener? Do you believe both, you and the surgeon, are in agreement about what outcome you can expect?

Will they perform the surgery in the least invasive manner possible? Will they force me to go under general anesthesia if there are other options available?

Question 4

According to the American Society of Aesthetic Plastic Surgery.

What's the most popular cosmetic surgery for men?

a. Face Lift
b. Tummy Tuck
c. Rhinoplasty (Nose reshaping)
d. Liposuction
e. Pectoralis implants

The answer is d. The most popular cosmetic surgery for men is liposuction.

Chapter 5

Tumescent Anesthesia

Tumescent anesthesia is a form of anesthesia invented by Dr. Jeffrey Klein, a dermatologist. We initially mentioned Dr. Klein in Chapter 3.

He came up with a dilute solution of fluid to help control pain, both during and after surgery. In addition, his solution also helped minimize any bleeding during surgery.

In other words, it is a solution which allows a doctor to perform surgery with virtually no blood loss and without having to go under general anesthesia.

In my opinion, this is one of the most significant advancements in cosmetic surgery. How amazing is that? We can now perform surgery without having to have to be sedated or having to go on a breathing machine. I, also, believe we should always perform surgery on patients in the least invasive manner whenever possible.

What kind of procedures can be done under local or tumescent anesthesia?

Despite how great I think tumescent anesthesia is, it cannot be used for all types of surgeries. There are times where general anesthesia is the safest way for the patient.

In our office, we do breast augmentations under local anesthesia. We also use tumescent anesthesia to perform liposuction alone or with fat transfer. Fat transfer is when we remove fat out from one area and place it in another area. We will go over fat transfer in Chapter 8.

There are also less invasive types of tummy tucks we perform in our office operating rooms without the need to go to sleep.

Will it hurt if I don't go to sleep?

It's impossible to tell anybody that they are not going to feel anything when they have surgery under tumescent anesthesia. Just by the virtue of the fact that they are awake, there are going to feel some sensations.

In general, the most uncomfortable part of tumescent anesthesia, similar to the part when you go to the dentist, is when the pain relief medicine is being injected.

I have had liposuction under tumescent anesthesia. (Yes! You read it correctly. I sure did! Dr. Owens performed liposuction of my abdomen and love handles in November 2017.) I can say I felt some burning while the medicine was being injected and that was it. Once that part was completed, I had no more discomfort.

Dr. Klein's solution has really great anesthetic properties and patients usually tolerate the surgery extremely well. Many patients will tell me they experienced a lot of pulling and tugging but that is all they felt. Some women have even compared it to having a cesarean section.

One thing I find very interesting is that occasionally I have to do a breast augmentation under general anesthesia for a multitude of different reasons. Maybe the person has a certain health problem and for that reason we have to have it done in the hospital rather than done in our office operating room system.

Those patients, of course, are completely asleep and don't feel anything while they are having the surgery. But as soon as they wake up from the general anesthesia, they are in more pain and discomfort than anything that typically goes on during our tumescent or local anesthesia surgeries.

I can tell you from my experience and from what I have gone through with both of these different types of anesthesia is that generally the entire process is a better experience for the patient under local or tumescent anesthesia compared to general anesthesia.

Can you talk me through a typical tumescent anesthesia case?

For our typical breast augmentation, the protocol starts the night before. The evening before surgery the patient will take a muscle relaxer and a sleeping pill to help them rest that evening. It is very important for them to get a good night's rest before surgery.

On the day of surgery, about an hour or two before the surgery is scheduled to begin, they take a pain pill and an additional sleeping pill. Most patients will experience a very relaxed feeling at that point.

When it is time to have surgery, the patient will walk themselves to the operating room to start the numbing process. During the procedure, the patient and I will talk about what sensations to expect.

Depending on how long the surgical case is, we will then discuss whatever topics come up or even sing. Yes, I sing! We usual have music playing in the operating room.

Whenever a song we really like comes on, I will always sing, and the patient typically laughs at me because I don't know the actual lyrics to any songs. There have even been times the patient will sing along with me and we actually sing a duet together. I swear this is true!! You can even ask my surgery assistant. They will tell you this has happened more than a few times.

Why do some surgeons only put patients to sleep to have surgery?

Doing surgery under tumescent or local anesthesia is something a surgeon must be trained to do. As surgeons, we all tend to do a lot of what we are trained to do and there are many doctors that once they receive training, stick with what they were taught and do not veer from that.

Then there are some doctors, like myself, who always want to find out if there are better and safer surgical procedures for their patients.

In essence, the reason doctors do not use tumescent or local anesthesia is because they can't, or they have not been trained.

When I first began doing cosmetics in 2006 it was kind of new to do these types of procedure, under this type of anesthesia. During my first consultations, I would spend a lot of time helping my patients understand the benefits of tumescent anesthesia.

It has now been many years since those first consultations. Now, I get patients who travel many hours to see me because doctors in their areas will only use general anesthesia or high-dose intravenous sedation.

Question 5

Who was the inventor of Tumescent Anesthesia?

a. Dr. Jeffrey Klein
b. Dr. John Gonzalez
c. Dr. Seuss
d. Dr. Dre
e. Dr. McDreamy

The answer is a. Dr. Jeffrey Klein was the inventor of Tumescent Anesthesia.

Chapter 6

Breast Implants

Saline or silicone? That is the question I hear the most from patients when they come in for a breast augmentation consult. The truth is there isn't a right or wrong answer to this question.

Let me give you my two cents about saline or silicone. There are two times I generally recommend silicone implants for patients, even though, the vast majority of women will do fine with saline implants.

Women who start off with less breast tissue to begin with or who have very thin skin, in my opinion, do better with silicone. A silicone implant feels more like natural breast tissue and there tends to be less rippling.

Rippling is when a person can see the shape or feel the implant through the skin. Rippling is not dangerous, so it is not a safety issue. However, some women do not like the way it looks.

So, for very thin, small breasted patients, I suggest silicone, if at all possible. Silicone implants cost a little bit more than saline implants so that also could possibly determine your choice. Either way, saline or silicone is fine. Most of my patients choose saline implants.

What is the best size breast implant for me?

I always like to ask patients what cup size they think they are now and what cup size they would like to be after surgery.

The reason I ask this is so that I can have a general idea of what it is they are thinking when they are considering these procedures.

For example, most women will come to me and they will tell me that they want to be a full C. I remember coming home talking to my wife about that and she says that what they truly mean is they want to be a D cup, but they are too embarrassed to say that because a D sounds so big. See! I told you I speak "Women".

I always remind my patients that there is no such thing as a full C cup and that every bra manufacturer is very different. Manufacturers use different type of standardizations for their cup sizes, so you may wear a C-cup in one brand and a D-cup in another.

Asking the question affords me the opportunity to listen to you and allows me to get a better idea of what type of results you are looking for.

Once I perform a physical exam on the patient and do chest wall measurements, I can determine what size implant I can place that best suits and matches your desired outcome.

From experience, I can tell you the average size implant I place in most women is around 400cc. However, I have placed implants as small as 230cc to as high as 750cc.

Should I have my breast implants placed over or under the muscle?

I place 99% percent of all implants under the muscle. The reason for placing them under the muscle is you get a lot better coverage of the implant by placing it under the pectoralis muscle.

What I mean is women who have thinner breast tissue will just have a little bit more tissue between the skin and the implant if it is placed under the muscle. Therefore, it is less likely to have the fake feeling women do not like that sometimes happens with saline implants.

The other reason from placing the implant under the muscle is that since you move your arms around a lot that will cause the implants to move. They are less likely to scar into place and get hard when they move around the pocket.

So, for the vast majority of women, I would recommend implants under the muscle.

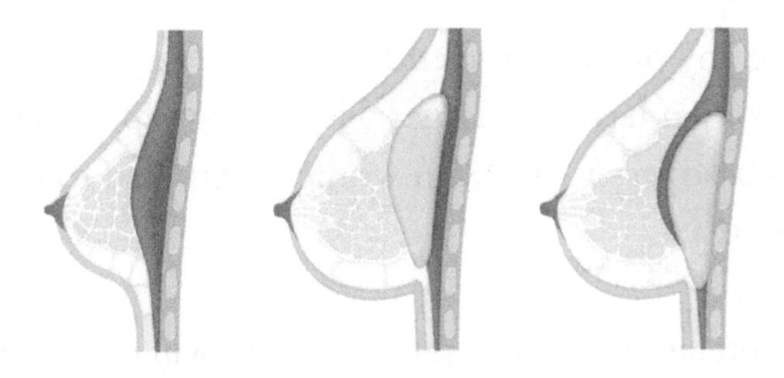

Where should the incision be placed for a breast augmentation?

There are a lot of different places the incision can be placed for just a basic breast augmentation. Breast implants can be placed through the peri areolar area (around the nipple), the axilla (armpit), through the belly button, or through an inframammary incision.

I would tell you that in our practice we mostly use the inframammary incision. That is when the incision is in the crease of the breast.

I prefer this incision for a couple of reasons. I think that from a cosmetic standpoint, it looks best. If there is a scar in the crease of the breast, then, the only way to see it is to lift the breast and look underneath.

Also, I find in my experience, that because we are not disrupting any of the nerve endings where milk ducts are located women have less issues with losing nipple sensitivity. There are also less issues with women who plan to breastfeed in the future.

There are not many surgeons who will do the incision in the armpit or the belly button. Those options are reserved for patients who really do not want to have a scar on their breasts at all.

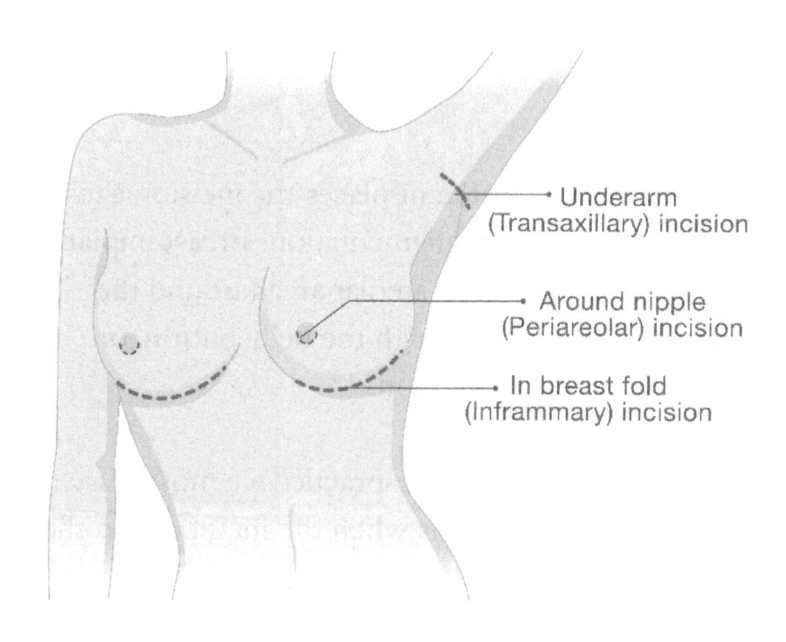

Can I breastfeed after getting breast implants?

We know that there is no harm to you or to the baby if you choose to breastfeed if you have implants. However, some women may find it to be a more difficult to breastfeed.

Regardless which type of incision is used, it is important to understand that by just placing an implant in the breast, some disruption of the milk ducts will occur.

How do I know if I need a breast lift?

We decide whether somebody needs a breast lift by determining where their nipple is in relation to the crease of the breast.

If you wanted to try a test at home to determine if a breast lift is right for you, take a pencil and place it underneath the crease of your breasts and then look in the mirror.

If the pencil is higher than your nipple, you most likely would benefit from a breast lift. This is a general rule of thumb and just a quick test you can do at home. *We would do a more thorough examination and discuss further during your consultation.*

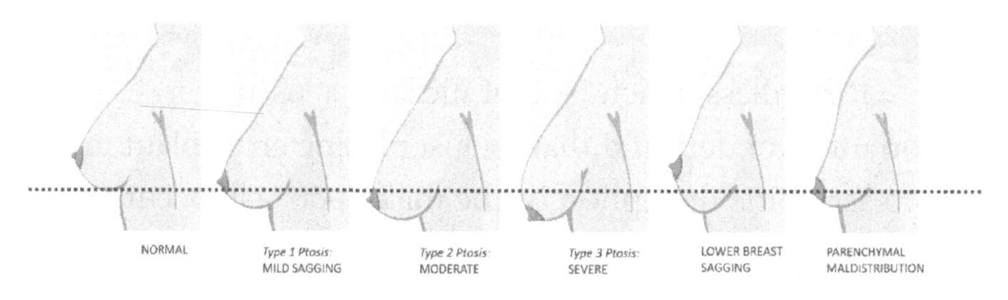

Will I lose nipple sensitivity?

Many patients will describe a change in nipple sensitivity after cosmetic breast surgery, but it typically returns to normal over time.

What if an implant ruptures?

If a saline implant ruptures, you will most likely notice it immediately because your breast will deflate. The good news is the saline we use to fill the implants is the same fluid you see in the IV bags when somebody goes in the hospital. We know this solution is perfectly safe and will be absorbed by your body.

Since there are no health risks with a deflated saline implant, there is no medical need to have it removed or exchanged. However, most patients do not like the appearance of having one breast smaller than the other, so they choose to have it exchanged for a new implant.

It is a little bit trickier to find a ruptured silicone implant. Since the implant is made of a gel, it does not leak out like a saline implant would. A ruptured silicone implant usually is only detected during a breast MRI or mammogram. Silicone implants are made of a cohesive gel and is often described as a Gummy Bear implant.

Both forms of implants have been studied extensively and are considered to be safe by the FDA.

Can breast implants burst if they are squeezed too hard?

I have never seen a breast implant burst from just being squeezed. The times I have seen an implant leak it usually is the result of a faulty valve or a defect in the implant shell. Unfortunately, implants can rupture during car accidents or sometimes if a woman is a victim of domestic violence or physical abuse.

But for normal run-of-the-mill activity, breast implants should not burst.

How often do I need to replace my breast implants?

There is not one correct answer. I have heard five years. I have heard seven years. I have heard ten years. I can tell you if your implants are not giving you any problems, then they do not need to be replaced.

My wife has had her breast implants for about seventeen years now and she has no problems with her breast. I have no intentions of changing them unless they leak.

I think some people get the idea implants need to be changed out is because they only have a ten-year manufacturer's warranty. I tell my patients if you have a car and your warranty is out on your car you don't just go ahead and sell the car. You just know that if anything happens it is not covered by the warranty anymore.

Question 6

According to the American Society of Aesthetic Plastic Surgery.

What is the most popular cosmetic surgery for women?

a. Cosmetic breast surgery
b. Liposuction
c. Tummy tuck
d. Face lift
e. Brazilian Butt Lift (BBL)

The answer is a. The most popular cosmetic surgery for women is cosmetic breast surgery

Chapter 7

Liposuction

Liposuction surgery consists of putting small holes in the areas where we want to remove fatty tissue. We place tubes through the holes and suck out the unwanted fat. This procedure really helps with the fatty tissue that you can pinch under the skin.

We all have that uncle in our families with a "big pot belly". You remember how hard his belly is, right? You could barely really pinch anything, and it is also hard as a rock. Well, unfortunately, that is somebody who liposuction is not going to help at all because of the type of fat that is.

LIPOSUCTION

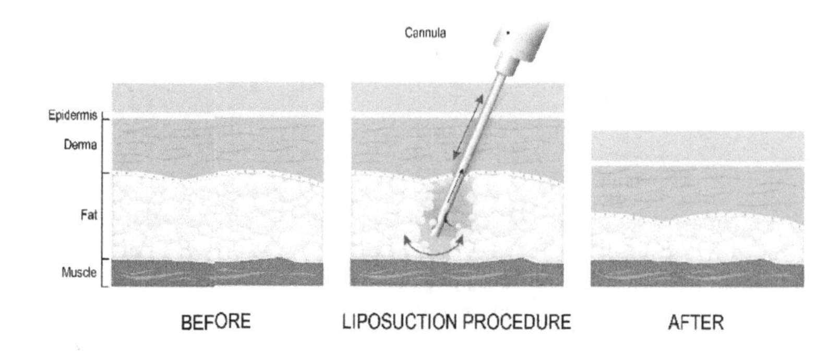

<u>Still not sure if liposuction is a good option for you? Call the office at (337) 785-2006 for your free consultation.</u>

Is liposuction a good way to lose weight?

Liposuction is a horrible way to lose weight. What you really should do is be at a steady weight before considering liposuction. The closer a person is to their ideal body weight the better the candidate for liposuction.

I would not say it is absolutely necessary to be a small person, but if you think of doing liposuction as a way to lose weight, you really are making a mistake.

I suffer from weight issues myself so believe me, when I say I share your pain and frustration. Doing liposuction as a way to lose weight will leave you disappointed.

The best thing to do if you have a weight issue is to develop healthy eating habits and increase your physical activity. When you get to a smaller size and have maintained your weight, then it would be a good time to consider getting cosmetic surgery.

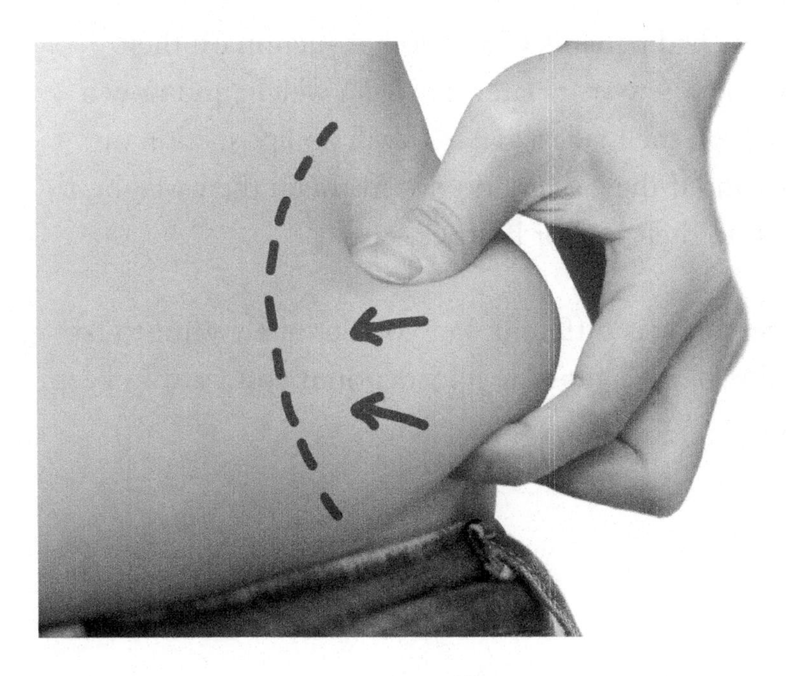

How long will the effects of liposuction last?

As long as you maintain your current weight, the results of liposuction are permanent. We are born with a certain amount of fat cells, and once those fat cells are gone, those fat cells are gone forever.

The cells we leave behind can swell up again so if we do not monitor our eating and gain weight it does have to go somewhere. I have found that if a person gains weight after having liposuction the areas that have not had liposuction tend to get bigger.

I have had patients who I do liposuction on their abdomen and a few years later they gain weight and now it comes back on their sides. Then, I will do liposuction on their sides and if they, again, do not maintain their weight, it may return to their legs or buttocks.

Everybody is different, but you definitely want to try to maintain your weight after liposuction if you want to keep your results.

Will liposuction improve cellulite?

Liposuction will not improve cellulite. There are really only a few things out there on the market today that can permanently improve cellulite. However, liposuction is definitely not one of them.

As a matter of fact, liposuction can actually worsen the appearance of cellulite.

Which body areas can be treated with liposuction?

The most common areas that we treat with liposuction are the belly, thighs (both outer and inner thighs), arms, and what I call the, back and hips area. Those are the typical areas. As a matter of fact, any area above the muscle layer where fatty tissue deposits exist can technically be liposuctioned.

Some atypical areas we can perform liposuction on are the chin, breasts, knees, bra-fat area, and the buffalo hump where some patients have a large fatty deposit where the neck meets the upper back.

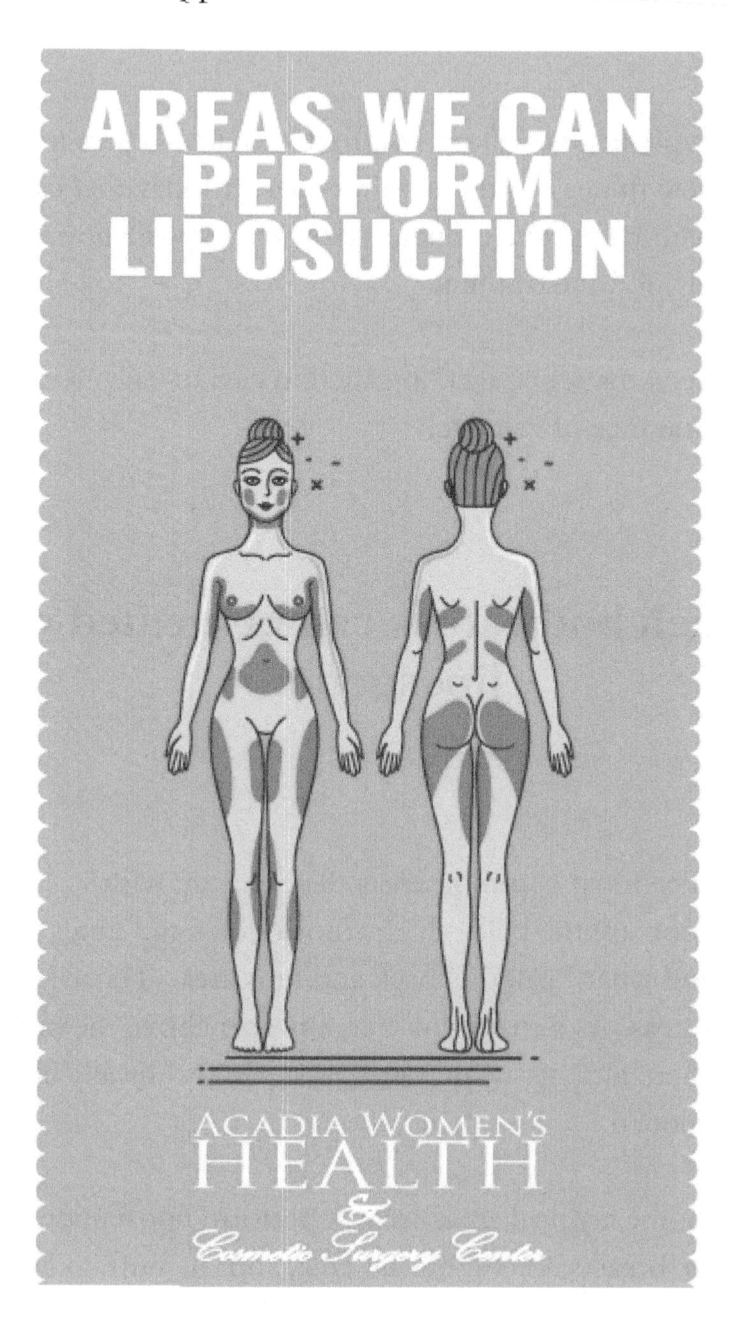

When can I see results from liposuction?

Some liposuction results initially can be seen within the first couple of days after surgery.

After the first few days, some swelling sets in. At this time, you may acquire lymphedema, which will give you a lumpy bumpy appearance to the areas that were lipoed.

The swelling usually goes away around six weeks after surgery. For some patients, it may take months to get the final results.

What is the most fat that can be removed by liposuction?

There are some safety limitations on how much fat can be taken out at one time if we are doing the procedure in an outpatient setting.

In my practice, the limit that we can take out at one time is four liters, which is nearly nine pounds of fatty tissue. I will tell you that getting close to nine pounds is pretty tough, even if I try to remove as much fat as possible.

The amount of fat I remove at one time for most patients usually depends on the area. For example, it is typical to remove about two to three pounds from the abdomen. For the back and love handles, maybe somewhere around three or four pounds of fat is average.

Will I have loose skin after liposuction?

Whether you will have a lot of loose skin after liposuction, will depend on your body. If you have good skin elasticity, the excess skin should retract and tighten over time.

If somebody has really flaccid or thin skin or there are stretch marks in areas we are liposuctioning, I will tell the patient they may have a bigger issue with loose skin. The truth is, however, even seeing stretch marks does not always mean there will be excessive looseness after liposuction. So, the real answer is that it just depends.

The two areas more prone to looseness after liposuction are the lower abdominal area and the inner thighs. It is my job during the consultation to ask the right questions and listen to the patient's desired outcome. I make sure I know what outcome they are looking for.

Occasionally, I will get somebody who I do not think is a great candidate for liposuction because I am worried about their skin issues. They tell me their main goal after surgery is to just feel better in their clothes and have them fit nicer. They are not worried about getting in a bikini and having everyone look at their body. They are not worried about being seen without their clothes on. They just want their clothes to fit them right and they do not want to go through the more invasive procedures to address the loose skin.

As long as we both, the patient and I, have a good understanding of the post-operative outcome, we will go forward with liposuction.

Question 7

True or False

Plastic Surgeons are the only qualified doctors capable of performing cosmetic surgery?

False. Plastic surgeons would like you to believe this is true, but it is not true. Many General Surgeons, Ob/Gyn's, and ENT's have the training and experience to perform cosmetic surgery.

Chapter 8

Tummy Tucks

A lot of people do not know the difference between liposuction and a tummy tuck. I will tell you that until I was in medical school I did not know the difference either. So, do not feel bad if you are not exactly sure.

Liposuction is where we make little holes and we suck out fatty tissue from skin that we can pinch. A tummy tuck is where we cut loose fatty skin out and remove it.

During a tummy tuck, we usually go ahead and tighten your abdominal muscles, the area many people describe as their six pack. Tightening these muscles, especially for women whose muscles have been separated and weakened from pregnancy, is very important. Because the loose abdominal skin is removed, a new opening for the belly button must be created.

The final result usually leaves a patient with two incisions; one in their lower half of their belly that goes across their abdomen and, another, around the belly button.

Do I need a full or a mini tummy tuck?

There are different types of tummy tucks. The one I described earlier is considered a full or traditional tummy tuck. It is when we remove a lot of skin from below the belly button and make a new opening for the belly button.

Some people who just may have some skin elasticity issues and only have a little bit of muscle weakness in the lower part of their belly may just need a mini tummy tuck.

This procedure does not require the belly button to be moved. A mini tummy tuck will result in a smaller scar in the lower abdomen and no scar around the belly button.

I, also, do a procedure we call a Brazilian Tummy Tuck. This is a procedure first described by Dr. Avelar, a cosmetic surgeon in Brazil. Liposuction is performed, and loose skin is removed, leaving the muscles intact.

A Brazilian Tummy Tuck is done in the office under tumescent anesthesia and is best for patients who do not need the abdominal muscle tightening of a traditional tummy tuck.

Determining who is a better candidate for which procedures really just requires a consultation to examine the patient. We do have a lot of patients who will call on the phone and ask how much tummy tucks cost.

My staff is always leery giving out prices over the telephone because they are not sure what type of surgery would be appropriate for them. So, we will ask them to come in for a free consultation.

Still not sure whether you are a better candidate for liposuction or one of the different types of tummy tucks? Stop spending hours online looking for the answer. Just call our office at (337) 785-2006 and come see me and we can decide together.

Will a tummy tuck help with stretch marks?

The answer to that is yes and no. All of the stretch marks in the area of the skin that is being removed will be gone after a tummy tuck. But if you have stretch marks in the area of skin we are not removing, they will remain.

Having said that, I find most women have the majority of their stretch marks in the lower abdominal area which is the area usually removed during a tummy tuck.

I plan to have more children. Should I get a tummy tuck?

It is not my place to tell you to have or not to have a tummy tuck if you plan to have more children. However, I would not recommend having a tummy tuck if you plan to have more children.

I believe a tummy tuck is a type of surgery you only want to have once. Remember a tummy tuck involves tightening up abdominal muscles and removing loose skin.

If someone has a tummy tuck and then years later they decide to have a baby, all of that area we tightened will get stretched out again. They are going to most likely be disappointed. At that point, they will most likely want to have another tummy tuck.

For patients that would like to improve their bodies with cosmetic surgery but are not sure if they are done bearing children, there is an alternative. Liposuction is something a lot more reasonable for patients who would like to improve the contour of their bodies but are not done having children.

It is not uncommon to perform liposuction on the same area more than once.

Can exercise tighten loose skin without a tummy tuck?

No. With just exercising, there is no way to tighten loose skin. Exercising is excellent for your health and to help you lose weight.

However, if you lose a lot of weight, you may even worsen the loose skin. The reason it may get worse is because fatty tissue sometimes bulks up the skin and when the fat goes away, the skin gets even looser.

Question 8

True or False

An abdominoplasty (tummy tuck) is an effective way to remove loose skin and stretchmarks.

True. Having a tummy tuck is a great way to remove excess skin and stretchmarks. Not to mention it also helps tightening up your abdominal muscles.

Chapter 9

Fat Transfers

Fat transfer is where we take fat out from one area of the body and then transfer it to another area the of the body. It involves performing liposuction on an area and then placing it back in another area that may need more fat. For some people, this may sound bizarre.

Those not familiar with fat transfer, may ask "Who would want to add fat to their bodies?". You have to realize what society considers beautiful has evolved over the years.

Everyone is familiar with the expression "curves in all the right places". Well, those right places may require removing fat in some areas of the body and enhancing other areas with that same fat. This often requires both liposuction to remove the fat and fat transfer to enhance another area.

We perform many fat transfers on our patients. Fat can be transferred to the buttocks, face and hands.

What is a BBL?

A BBL, or as it is more commonly known as a Brazilian Butt Lift, is where we take fat, usually from the back and sides, and transfer it to the buttocks. It is a procedure which seems to be taking America by storm.

It first became popular amongst my African American and Latina patients in 2014, but now seems to have crossed ethnic lines and has become one of my most requested procedures.

Many patients will request fat be removed from their abdomen and transferred to the buttocks, rather than from their back and sides.

Fat can truly be taken from anywhere and transferred to the buttocks, but part of giving a woman a shapelier butt is to shape the lower back and hips to improve the contour. This is accomplished by performing liposuction on the lower back and hips. Then, by injecting the fat removed from those areas to the buttocks we are able to increase the size and projection of the butt.

Can someone else donate fat to me for a Brazilian butt lift?

No, the fat has to come from you, because just like any other organ your body would reject it and may make you extremely ill if it came from someone else.

Theoretically if you had an identical twin you could use their fat but even then, there are safety issues to consider and it should not be done.

I do run across patients who are too thin and don't have enough fat to remove and transfer to their buttocks. In those instances, I may encourage a patient to gain 10-15 pounds or to consider buttock implants.

How long do Brazilian butt lift results last?

In my experience about 65 to 75 percent of the fat we transfer survives. There are many factors to consider and this number can vary considerably from person to person.

For fat to survive after transfer it must get blood supply from the surrounding tissue. Once the fat gets blood supply then it is permanent and will be just like any other fat you have in your body.

What is the recovery time for a Brazilian Butt Lift?

The recovery time for a BBL depends on the type of work you do. Most women who have desk jobs take off about three to four days.

Dr. Owens performed liposuction on my abdomen on a Saturday and I returned to work the following Monday.

The BBL recovery is a little different, however, because we ask patients not to sit directly on their buttocks for two to three weeks after the fat transfer. If they sit directly on their buttocks, they will displace some of the fat we transferred, which may inhibit the blood supply to the newly transferred fat.

The goal is for the fat to get new blood supply, for it to stay where it was placed and be permanent. Additionally, sitting may shift some of the fat to other places affecting the improved contour we are trying to achieve.

If sitting is a necessary part of your job, there are some products on the market patients can purchase who need to return to sitting sooner than the recommended two to three weeks.

Can I inject fat into my breast instead of using implants?

Patients will often wonder and ask me that if fat can be transferred to all these other places, can't we just transfer it to my breast instead of having a breast augmentation. My answer is yes you can transfer fat to your breasts, but I do not recommend it.

The reason I do not recommend it in my practice is because I think breast implants are a better option. I think this is confusing for patients because one of the most common places to transfer fat is to the buttocks and you rarely hear people say they have had buttock implants.

When we are looking to augment the size of a woman's buttocks, one of the options is buttocks implants. However, I will tell you that the complication rate from buttocks implants tend to be a lot higher than seen with breast implants.

There are a few reasons for this. Since the buttock area is near a place where there is a lot of bacteria, buttock implants tend to have more infections and wound breakdowns.

On the other hand, breasts implants have less of these issues. I think it is the safer and better option to place a breast implant to enhance the size of the breasts instead of fat transfer.

Question 9

According to the American Society of Aesthetic Plastic Surgery.

What percentage of all cosmetic surgeries are performed on men?

a. 8%
b. 18%
c. 28%
d. 38%
e. 98%

The answer is a. 8% of all cosmetic surgeries are performed on men.

Chapter 10

How Can I Make My Face Look Younger?

I get this question often and there are a lot of things that you can do to help you look younger. Everyone wants to slow down the aging process.

The most important thing is to take good care of your skin and be proactive. Do not wait until you start to see a lot of wrinkles to start paying attention your skin.

If you come from a family where you know the skin elasticity is poor, you need to start sooner than later.

It is never too late or too early to start caring for your skin but once in your mid-twenties, extra care should be taken. It does not mean I would run and do a facelift just because I saw one wrinkle. I think this is the time to come up with a strategy for your future face.

It is always good to go for the low hanging fruit first and it does not get any easier than staying out of the sun. Sun can cause significant skin damage.

Wearing a wide brimmed hat and applying sunscreen are minimum recommendations when going outside. Using a good skin care line is also important.

Acadia Women's Health has developed a skin care line for all women and men. It is called The Real OG Skin Care. It was designed with the Louisiana patient in mind.

Between the heat and excessive humidity, we experience in the South, it can really wreak havoc on a person's skin. Taking good care of your skin is paramount. Many patients have commented that they like it even more than the Obagi line.

Head to our website www.acadiawomenshealth.com/shop or come to the office to get started on improving your skin.

What is Botox and how does it work?

Botox is medical-grade dilute botulism toxin. That may sound scary, but it is not. The toxin is a substance which paralyzes muscles and, when used in dilute doses, can prevent wrinkles in those areas. For example, there are a lot of patients that can see two vertical wrinkles right above their nose when they frown or when they contract the muscles in their brow.

Overtime, the creases get deeper and deeper. Other troublesome areas are the crow's feet (the area on the sides of your eyes) and the area on the forehead when you lift up and raise your eyebrows.

When we inject Botox in those areas, it will paralyze those muscles for a short period of time allowing those wrinkles to go away. Botox lasts for about three to four months and is a procedure you must upkeep.

I would not suggest having Botox once and then never doing it again. Botox is something we recommend doing regularly and usually becomes part of most people's skin care regiment.

Why do some places sell BOTOX for so cheap and others are more expensive?

I cannot speak for everybody, but I can tell you what we do in our practice. We charge patients $12 a unit and we buy Botox directly from the manufacturer. We buy it directly from the company who makes it, Allergan.

It happens to be the same company we buy our breast implants from. We buy so many breast implants and Botox from Allergan that we receive the best prices available. In other words, we pay the lowest price offered from the company who makes Botox.

Our cost for Botox is about $7 a unit so I am always surprised when I see other offices advertise $6 or $8 a unit for Botox. *It makes me wonder if they are diluting their Botox too much or if they are purchasing their products through Mexico.*

It is not uncommon for me to receive faxes and email requests to purchase Botox for extremely low prices, but this particular Botox is coming from Mexico or other areas. I refuse to purchase Botox from other countries.

I know with **100%** certainty the Botox used in my office has been bought directly from Allergan and is going to be injected by a doctor who is trained in Botox, not a nurse or aesthetician. I can't speak for any other practice or doctor; on how they mix their Botox or where they get their Botox from.

What I can tell you is in our practice we follow the manufacturer's recommendations and we buy it directly from the manufacturer. ***Buyer beware of Botox less than $12 a unit!!!***

What to expect after a Botox injection?

For the first 20 minutes after a Botox injection the little spots injected will look like mosquito bites. Generally, within an hour or two, that goes away.

We tell our patients to refrain from physical exertion for the first 4 hours after injections because we do not want the medicine to migrate into other areas we did not inject. After a few days, those muscles become paralyzed temporarily.

Then you will start to notice that your skin will take a shinier appearance and those wrinkles will either fade away completely or will be a lot less noticeable than before.

Of course, your results will depend on how deep your lines and wrinkles were before we started.

How do Juvederm or Restylane work?

Dermal fillers are other products on the market to improve wrinkles. Botox works by paralyzing muscles and it works well for the areas that we described earlier, essentially the upper part of the face.

The lower part of the face like the frown lines or the area we call the nasal labial fold which run from your nostril all the way to the side of your mouth, tend do a lot better with fillers.

The two main fillers we use are Restylane and Juvederm. By injecting these fillers directly into the wrinkle causes the skin to plump up and the lines and wrinkles become less noticeable.

Juvederm and Restylane injections tend to last about six to nine months. Fillers are something which requires maintenance and should be done on a regular basis.

What to expect after a filler injection?

Fillers can leave a little bit of bruising in the areas injected but can be easily covered up with some makeup. There may also be some tenderness and soreness in those areas, as well.

Question 10

According to the American Society of Aesthetic Plastic Surgery.

On average, how old are people who get cosmetic surgery?

a. 21
b. 31
c. 41
d. 51
e. 101

The answer is c. The average age of a person having cosmetic surgery is 41.

Chapter 11

I'm Ready, What Next?

I hope you have found this book useful. Cosmetic surgery has become part of the American culture and is here to stay. With all of the changes happening in healthcare, these are exciting times for patients.

Thanks to the internet and patient demand for more transparency, there has never been more information readily available to the public. With all of this new information, it has become nearly impossible to decipher what is true and what is "Fake News".

Finding a reliable trustworthy source is more difficult than it ever has been. I hope I can become that trusted source for you. Remember this process is about YOU, the patient, *not* about the doctor.

We have gone over the most common cosmetic procedures. You now know more about breast augmentations, liposuction and tummy tucks than most people in the world today.

You have been waiting your entire life for this. It is time to finally get closer to having the body you have been dreaming of. What else is holding you back? What are you waiting for? There will never be a perfect time? So, why not now? Once you do it, you will wonder why you waiting so long?

Find a doctor who is a better listener than speaker. If you go into a consultation and the surgeon is doing all of the talking, I suggest you walk out and come see me. I will do my best to listen and communicate with you always. All of my cosmetic surgery patients receive my person cell phone number and I hear from them regularly. Hope to see you soon!

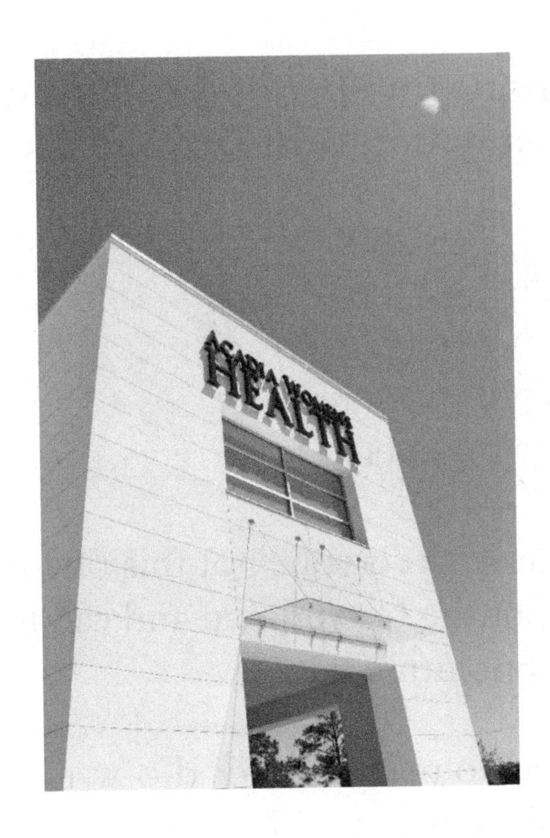

Visit our website at
www.acadiawomenshealth.com
or call our office at (337) 785-2006 to schedule a free consultation with me.

527 Odd Fellows Road Suite B

Crowley, LA 70526

Question 11

What phone number do I call to schedule a free consultation with Dr. Gonzalez?

a. (337) 785-2006
b. (337) 785-2006
c. (337) 785-2006
d. (337) 785-2006
e. (337) 785-2006

My guess is everyone got this one right!!! Now put the book down and call to make your appointment.

No, no, no really. P-u-t d-o-w-n t-h-e b-o-o-k a-n-d c-a-l-l.